Secrets To Unleashing Your

Inner Motivation Fierce Factor

90 ~ Day Motivational

Renatta McCoy - Baker

I give Honor and Thanks to God who continues to keep me in his Master Plan…..

~Renatta

'Born again'

~Passion~

Passion is what moves you to persevere at
something despite fear, unhappiness or pain.

This book is designed to unleash your Inner Motivation Fierce Factor (IMFF). Yes another cute and friendly acronym to add to your alphabet soup. You will master and overcome the common excuses, negative thoughts and sabotaging mindset blocking you from your desires, goals and realizing your aspirations. In just as little as 90 days you will have uncovered your inner voice to coach yourself to success in every aspect of your life.

Each day will build your confidence needed to conquer fear, self-doubt, procrastination and all your reasons & excuses that have formed the

negative associations and patterns
of a poorly trained mindset.

Do you realize you can attract &
obtain anything you train your brain
to accomplish? So many people
struggle year end and year out and
can never put their finger on why life
is not working out for them. They
want to change their life but really
don't understand the mechanics
behind how change meets the rubber
in the road. They dismiss it as not
having enough education or not
being smart enough even thinking
God has cursed them for some
reason. Stop right this moment if
this is you, I want you to stop
reading and think about the negative
picture you have painted in your

mind over the years. It is never too late to start a new bright colorful outlook on life.

In order to get the most Life has to offer you must take full control of your mind. Stop allowing life to give you the leftovers.

You are the master chef of your universe. The universe is here to serve you! So create your 5 course meal and include dessert. Dig deep and settle in on learning how to master the power of mind over all matter. Conquer your mind and change your circumstances, your life, your world.

Are you ready to tap into your own greatness? Well what are you waiting for? Without further ado "Unleash your Inner Motivation Fierce Factor"!

Holistically Yours, *Coach Renatta*

"The Health Crusader"

| MOTIVATIONAL PRAYER |

Dear God why didn't you give me as much motivation as I have desire?

Isaiah: 40:29-31: He gives power to the faint, and to him who has no might he increases strength. Even youths shall faint and be weary, and young men shall fall exhausted; but they who wait for the LORD shall renew their strength; they shall mount up with wings like eagles; they shall run and not be weary; they shall walk and not faint. (NIV)

Galatians: 6:9: And let us not grow weary of doing good, for in due season we will reap, if we do not give up. (NIV)

Hebrews: 12:11: For the moment all discipline seems painful rather than pleasant, but later it yields the peaceful fruit of righteousness to those who have been trained by it. (NIV)

2 Timothy 1:7: For the Spirit God gave us does not make us timid, but gives us power, love and self-discipline (NIV)

Joshua 1:9: Have I not commanded you? Be strong and courageous. Do not be frightened, and do not be dismayed, for the LORD your God is with you wherever you go." (NIV)

Psalm 128:2: You will eat the fruit of your labor; blessings and prosperity will be yours. (NIV)

John 5:17: In his defense Jesus said to them, "My Father is always at his work to this very day, and I too am working." (NIV)

1 Corinthians 15:58: Therefore, my dear brothers and sisters, stand firm. Let nothing move you. Always give yourselves fully to the work of the Lord, because you know that your labor in the Lord is not in vain. (NIV)

| WHAT IS MOTIVATION? |

Derived from the Latin word
"MOVERE" translated: TO MOVE!

Internal and external factors that
stimulate desire and energy in
people to be continually persistent
with enthusiasm & positive thoughts,
to sustain a high level of interest &
focus in being committed to an idea
or cause, as to make a conscious
effort to attain goals and aspirations
in every area of life.

WHERE'S MY MOTIVATION?

The million dollar question! If only we could purchase motivation in a pill! We still would lose our motivation from time to time. It would never fail, we would become unmotivated at some point to not take the pill. We would abandon or dismiss the pill and use the excuse "I need an easier way to swallow it". Then set off to find it in a liquid form to guzzle it down the hatch. Many people view motivation as some fluke of nature sometimes we feel motivated and sometimes we don't. We pray to God to become more motivated in our spiritual walk, our health & wellness, our finances, our relationships.

We seek out motivation on book shelves in books (just like this one you're reading now!). We throw big money at the latest fancy smancy pants "New Year - New Me" challenges that promise to keep us more engaged than the year before. A ton of personal development groups pop up all over social media warning you not to dilly dally this year come join us Now! The potential and excitement of a New Year lures in the same faces with a few new motivationally challenge souls that seek to snatch the pebble from the coach's hand (the pebble symbolizing the motivation they seek). It all starts with the count down 5...4...3...2...1....the screams of "Happy New Year!!!"

We emerge on January 1st every year with so much hope and potential to finally catch our dreams after chasing them for years. We set out to go find the cutest planner of the year. You find the one, your favorite color with words that sparkle "If You Can Dream It! You Can Do It!" This one is for you this planner will make all of your goals come true this year. Off you go!! You open up to the very first page and scribble some goals deliberately in pencil because you're not even sure about what you just declared. Now you are ready to rock and roll. The only thing is you give yourself an unofficial, unspoken & unabashed grace period to get all of last's year's residual bad habits out of our system. As we silently try and convince ourselves to try it yet again with a big sigh and eye roll of "doubt", "disbelief", "don't wanna do's", the   "can't find the time" and "oh it didn't work before". Oh what fun to fill our planners with new goals & new project plans with generous timelines for completion! We revisit the same ole declarations we make each year to eat healthier, exercise more, reduce our stress, start our new business, go back to school, write that book or take that vacation so on and so forth.

The habitual Ready Set Go!
Then the days start to add up and
we don't hit our goals, we not only
fall short, we lay down and get
comfortable and prop the pillow into
our comfort zone of the "To be
completed list". We start hiding and
ducking from the personal trainer.
Our initial motivation to wear the
gym out has worn out. We figure we
can miss a few gym days hey what
the heck we got the rest of the year
to get it done. A few missed
workouts turn into a complete No-
show at the gym for months.

We send our accountability
partner's call to voicemail because
we dread the "what happened to
you" conversations about cancelled

plans. Wait, it gets worst, we reason
with lies that comfort us & keeps us
tied to those habitual bad habits.
Hummph! does this ring a bell to
anyone besides me? Maybe it's just
me, but I remember those days.

Motivation is one of the hardest
skills to cultivate, keep energized &
keep your enthusiasm high over
consecutive long periods of time.
Most often our motivation is very
much tied to our emotional and
physical state of being. It's really
that simply yet complicated at the
same time. Simply put we all have
our infamous comfort zone and we
do what we feel like doing most times
and anytime. Doing what we feel like
doing is warm and cozy like a hot cup

of pumpkin spice latte on a brisk fall day. Doing what we feel like doing is a strategy that has never worked in our best interest in the past but has become our "Modus Operandi".

Our source of motivation can come from various situations and circumstances in our lives. It can be tied to people, places and things that have inspired us to live more, dream bigger and go that extra mile. We all have different personal triggers that either gets us going or shuts us down.

Motivation can be tied to a traumatic experience or it can be birthed out of a desire to change something we feel deeply & strongly about in our souls. Or in a very narrow view, motivation can be more superficial in nature and we become unmotivated when our priorities in life have changed. People who are more tied to passionate soul stirring triggers are more likely to stay motivated longer to reach their goals versus people who are motivated by a less passion filled "Why".

The stronger our "Why," typically the fiercer our motivation is to continue on our path, task, goals and our dreams. Take a single mother who is working 2 jobs to keep food on the table and a roof over her and her children's head.

This mother's "Why" makes her immune to any excuses she could use to give up! Her "Why" is her reason! Her motivation is emotionally attached to the welfare of her children and this emotion is a very deep etched soul tie to her motivation.

So why does motivation start off as an avalanche pretty much a snow ball rolling down the mountain gaining momentum on its way down forming a huge ball of massive snow then all of a sudden it rolls back up the mountain losing snow on its ascent back up the mountain.

Ok what just happened here? Where did my big snowball of motivation go? In my animated analogy I wanted to convey how motivation is there one minute and gone the next second. We have all played the motivational musical chairs game.

The reason why our motivation comes and goes is because motivation is highest at the mere thought of achieving our goals. As that thought goes through our motivation lifecycle process, there are emotions and feelings that deeply impact our ability to continue to feel excited about the work that has to be done, to achieve the goals we have set. Then there is this thing called life, whew life whips up on us pretty good sometimes.

Inevitably, life will always happen & then there are always those old emotions and feelings we tuck deep underneath our best wardrobe that say "Hello" as soon as distractions ring our doorbell. As you welcome them all in to your "Pity Procrastination Party". This is one of the loneliest parties in the world. We dance to the beat of "We don't feel like it", "We are too tired", "Next week when I get paid", "Not now", and "I'm too busy". Our motivation takes a nose dive, slips, regresses, backslides, plays peek-a-boo, and downright leaves us hanging off of a cliff and tips it's hat

"Good Luck with that you're on your own!".

Do not feel bad if your motivation waxes and wanes it is the typical ebb and flow of life. To some extent it can be addressed with strategies and habits to support keeping your motivation balanced and actively working towards meeting your goals. However, it is beneficial to note if you struggle with some form of mental illness such as severe bouts of depression, anxiety any mental health issues you have been clinically diagnosed with. I strongly recommend the expertise of a professional medical doctor or psychologist to treat more severe cases of lack of motivation due to depression. *Disclaimer: this book is not intended to diagnose or treat any medical illness and should not be used in place or override your doctor's advice.

This book is intended to awaken your motivational giant to provoke real thought, mediation and unleash the power of your mind soul body. It is designed to give you a nudge, push and sometimes slap you back to the realities of your abilities to achieve your best life. If you want to be reminded of how great you are! Read this book!

This book gives you 100 days of gentle reminders that you are bigger than your biggest goal. This book is for all who not only dare to dream but dare to believe, try, work and accomplish so much more in life.

For 90 days and 10 additional bonus days, meditate expand and apply these daily inspirational insights to your current life aspirations.

Reach for this book when you need a little extra thumbs up, when your motivation is running low, when you need to get back on track with aligning what you said you would do and what you need to do!

It is my intent to reignite, provoke, engage, and mentally keep your motivation pot of water that you have put on the stove for tea from evaporating into thin air. We all have put some water on for a cup of tea and forgot about it and come back to a scorched pot with not even a drip drop of liquid. This is what happens to our motivation essentially we start out with a full pot of water and get distracted doing other things and have to put more water in the pot only this time we will not leave it unattended. It is the same for our motivation. We cannot allow our motivation to evaporate into thin air!   Constantly remind yourself of your goals daily. Keep a record of what you are doing to reach those goals you have set for yourself.

Viewing your daily progress is a good tool to keep your motivation levels high.

This book is not written from a clinical perspective so don't worry about being presented with mounds of studies and clinical reasons with grim statistics as to why you simply are "Duffing your Fluff" translation "Goofing your Greatness".

I don't want to give any spoiler alerts but let's just say you will be more informed and more motivated after reading this book.

There is even a small token for accomplishing your 100 days of "Secrets to Unleashing your Inner Motivation Fierce Factor" strong. You will have to read on to uncover the Secrets!!!

"What is my calling?"

We were all designed and purposed in life for God's unique plan! Our soul's connection to our creator is what drives our spirit. Many people spend a lifetime wondering about their purpose and calling in life. The soul seeks ultimate purpose!

When feelings of angst, desperation, despair, loneliness, anger, confusion, sadness and boredom set in, it is our conscious mind reminding us of our purpose waiting to be revealed. All of life's little nudges, pokes and aha moments exist to makes us tap into our inner being. It's easy to get lost in the enchanted forest of the world's perfect "Dream Life" beckoning you to join the crowd, fit in, sit pretty, don't question and just exist, and go with the program.

It takes deep self- awareness and an introspective view in order to uncover your life's purpose. Your purpose is and has always been with you. We have put on many layers of other people's thoughts and opinions for our lives. Our purpose is buried deep within us we are very removed from ourselves in so many ways that we don't even notice subtle hints or bang the drum clues about what inspires & free our souls

to contribute our part of our story
of this thing called "Life".

Instead of going with our intuition or
our gut feeling we defer to the court
of popular opinion which unfairly,
unjustly and without warrant judges
our soul by generic labels and ideals.
It is our God given responsibility to
find out what our purpose is and live
it out and express it fully. Motivated
people realize their purpose and
every thought and every action
supports the way they show up in
the world. Motivation influenced by
purpose fueled with intention and
drive brings dreams to reality.

Life is our road of purpose. We are
the vehicle on the road of Life.
Motivation is the gas to keep us
driving along purposely in life.
Passion is our ability to continue the
ride through all of life's rough
patches and not abandon our
journey for an easier road.

| MOTIVATIONAL TRAITS |

There is always the presumption of privilege associated with very successful people. Successful people who were not born into wealth are highly self-motivated individuals, which in a sense is a privilege. The people who manage to keep their motivation at very high levels at any given time and unapologetically max out what life has to offer. They also know living their highest quality of life requires a special set of skills to master the "The Art of Motivation". Every aspect of inspired living requires motivation to get there.

Motivated people tend to be very successful in many areas of life. They do not require hand holding or need to be coddled or cosseted and hit the ground bouncing in pursuit of their dream life. Navigating the sea of life requires a certain level of "Kick butt I don't need to know your name" later attitude. Are these people born with an extra motivational chromosome gene?

Is this why we struggle and they swim laps around our mindless behavior of procrastination and whimsical thoughts of pursuing a goal & lack luster attitudes at a getting-err-done by all means necessary mindset. Hey there may be some smoke from a burning bush to investigate with this one. The correlation between go-getters and an imaginary motivation gene, has not yet been corroborated via doctors or scientist to date. Too bad we can't jump on the "Woe is me" wagon and sign up for disability for not having this special go forth and be great gene. The good news is that we all can work on our motivational skills. So how motivated are you at this very moment on a scale of 1 to 10? Do you have a goal to lose a few pounds but continue to buy your favorite ice cream? Do people ask you over and over about a goal or dream you been yapping about over the years?

Maybe you've reached some of your goals but let some goals slide. Well allow this book to give you an extra dose of therapy to add to your little tool box of motivation.

Understanding what motivation is and how it works can be a bridge over the troubled waters of procrastination, the undercurrent of doubt and fear. We don't reach goals out of sheer desire. Goals are only realized with proper strategies and focus.

| MOTIVATION .VS. INSPIRATION |

Motivation Pushes
Inspiration Pulls

Inspiration simply put means "To be In Spirit". When we are inspired to do something we are not concerned about the end result it's more about fulfillment and contentment. Inspiration is a calling and is effortless. It is a feeling deep in our bones, also known as "Intrinsic Motivation".

Maybe you can sew or crochet all day long or maybe you love to cook, read to children, minister the word of God, walk dogs or care for newborns. We never have a problem doing the things we enjoy or indulging in our passions. However, we lose our motivation starring at that big pile of dishes in the sink after having so much fun baking the cake and even more fun eating it. It's very self-rewarding to see our pie rise in the oven; it does our heart good to bake a good tasting moist pound cake from scratch of which we are inspired by every cup of sugar, stick of butter and dash of vanilla that it takes to make it.

"Extrinsic Motivation" is when you are motivated by external pressures to avoid punishment or looking for a reward up front. When we are motivated by things we must do but do not find any pleasure in doing them. Cleaning the kitchen, or washing the dishes after cooking would be an example of extrinsic motivation.

Motivation is our push through towards specific results. Inspiration is our pull from within that does not require extrinsic motivation it's a natural inclination to do something without respect to an outcome. Motivation needs many things and inspiration can be a factor but does not always have to be the source.

Motivation is our inner fierce factor our make it or break it zeal to change our habits, reach our goals and endure life challenges.

In this life we need: breath, love, will, faith, mental toughness, purpose, direction, forgiveness, strength, hope, dreams, health, growth and we need motivation for all the aforementioned.

| 7 SECRETS TO MOTIVATION |

Thinking well and eating well goes a long way on your journey of motivation.

1: DARK CHOCOLATE:

Eat a few slabs of chocolate. Increase your dopamine level which is our feel good hormone. When we feel good we are more inclined to reach our goals

2: GO GREEN FOR YOUR GOALS:

The color green has been known to increase motivation levels. Get outdoors on a natural trail to meditate, change your screen saver to green, drink a green smoothie, and

wear green to give you an extra
push.

3: LIMIT YOUR ENTERTAINMENT:

Finding time is a common excuse. The fastest way to increase your motivation is to minimize your entertainment to specific times of the day. Social media can create huge sink holes in our motivation. Ensure you are implementing time restrictions on all social media.

4: ADOPT A MANTRA

A mantra is a word, verse or sound repeated to aid in concentration. Motivation does not filter through chaos. The more clear you are the stronger your ability to focus on completing your goals. Repeating a strong belief of affirmation in words or sound cultivates clarity and mental dexterity.

Practice moments of Zen, close your eyes visualize & repeat your mantra the energy will strengthen your motivation.

5: LISTEN TO MUSIC

The music, mind, & motivation connection is powerful. Music and mood are inherently connected. Music's energizing effects comes from its ability to engage the body's sympathetic nervous system. This activates our readiness or preparedness for challenges the body faces mentally, spiritually and physically. Music has repetitive melodic beats that synchronizes and stimulates our brain waves.

If you are feeling stuck and you need some extra motivation throw on your favorite track to get you going and keep you motivated.

6: BE FLEXIBLE

Be determined, steadfast and unmovable about your goals but flexible enough to reach them. Do not get weighed down on doing anything one specific way. Flexibility allows motivation to continue when we hit those detours along the way.

7: SLEEP TIGHT

Motivation lies in our rest. Getting
the proper amount of sleep each
night, adds breadth and longevity to
our motivation. A peaceful good
night's rest will give you fuel to
power your motivation to get those
task completed and your things to
do list done!
Rest Assured!

| 10 SECRETS TO MOTIVATION |

1: LOSE YOUR DISTRACTIONS!

Ever notice how quickly you lose focus when you have a million things going on? Multi-tasking can be the death of focus and motivation. There is a big connection between motivation (lack thereof) and a distracted mind. Never has there ever been a more distracted society than we presently live in. Years ago we could simply turn off the television or take the phone off the hook.

Oh brother now there is technology,
social media and smart phones,
videos, podcast, webinars, live
streaming it is a miracle we get
anything done these days. Learn
how to eliminate as many distractions
as possible to maintain your focus.
If this means taking a break from the
world and social networks and
notifications then you have to make
some serious deliberate adjustments
the world will survive without your
social network presence.

2: SEEK A MENTOR!

You need people who are doing
what it is that you aspire to do!
Mentors provide insight & guidance
that funnel your sheer enthusiasm
down the most productive roads to

success. They are great for keeping your feet to the fire and redirecting you back to your "Why". Many mentors are not born with silver spoons in their mouths so they can offer practical advice and strategies on how to get to your next level. Mentors know that mentoring keeps their motivational skill set sharp as well.   Always mentor up and not down. What I mean by this is do not find any ole body or people in the same boat as you, when the going gets tough you need that expert push for accountability.

Your mentor should be qualified and a few notches tighter than where your belt is currently buckled. So tighten up!

3: KEEP SOME GOALS A SECRET!

Shhhhhhush it!! You may be thinking why should I keep my goals & dreams a secret? Here is why I say don't share everybody your teeth until you are ready to bite. Sometimes you just have to learn that everybody will not support your journey. They can be a hindrance with negative talk or even try and convince you that maybe your dreaming way out of your league.

Sure going public or announcing a big goal could potentially give you some extra motivation because now you have put it out there for the world to see and judge. There is nothing like declaring in 30 days you will lose 60lbs now everybody is closely watching and scrutinizing your progress which could be a negative effect. Once you allow people in on your goals and dreams many will try and talk you down from the ledge with all your lofty goals. I have seen it plenty of times.

People mean well but are unconscious of their own faulty mindset. There are many people who never set big goals in their life and are not mentally mature enough to handle your bulls' eye target goals.

So keep it buttoned up until you have gotten pretty good footing on the slippery slope of public opinion.

4: STAY HEALTHY!

Huh? What does this have to do with your motivation you ask or you are thinking you need the motivation to get healthy. What happens as soon as we get sick? Of course our motivation gets the flu too & gets put on the injured reserve list. Now we have a good reason not to make it to the gym and take a break from our motivation too. While we are on the sick and shut in list we are forced into the immediate need of self-care and our focus shifts to a man down situation & our motivation goes A-wall. So you want to ensure that you are eating properly and getting your rest to circumvent losing any motivation momentum. Unfortunately, we all get sick it is a part of life, but you want to ensure you are taking great care to remain healthy. Our health is our foundation for all we do in this life.

5: DEVELOP MORNING & NIGHTIME RITUALS!

Trying to stay motivated and keep up with all the things we have to do on a daily basis can create huge motivational pot holes on our path. Highly motivated people know the importance of creating routines to support reaching goals in life. What does your night-time ritual look like?

Do you strategize and plan for waking up to a plan of action that allows you to be more effective and efficient throughout your day?

Does your bedtime habit create a chaos filled morning rush out of the door?

Our night time strategies are just as important as our morning routine.

Add structure to your night give yourself enough time to plan and relax to ensure your mornings are powered with purpose.

6: CREATE A VISION DREAM BOARD!

Vision boards have been all the rage in the recent years. A vision board is a pictorial collection of your goals and dreams that you create to keep you motivated and front and center of your goals. Many people find vision boards very helpful as some of us are visually stimulated. And they are fun to create. There are some people who prefer writing their goals down in the form of a list this is a different type of vision board for those who prefer wording as opposed to pictures. Your vision board should be strategically placed where you can see if many times a day. Create a vision board for your home and office.

Mediate on your vision board daily! Seeing your goals visually standout jumps into your conscious and subconscious mind which forms an indelible impression in the mind. Vision boards are great reminders of what we want out of life. I know they are called vision boards and for good reason however, be mindful to include more than just material things on your dream board like images that inspire feeling.
Our dream board should evoke our motivation.

7: REWARD YOURSELF!

Learn how to recognize and celebrate small victories. Rewarding yourself for the progress you make along the way can be just the motivation boost you need. Don't forget to treat yourself good you are working on being better, doing better and feeling better. If you have kept up your daily habits for a week give yourself a gold star. If you are exercising to lose weight and lost a few pounds go shopping for a new dress.

You do not have to wait until you have finally reached a goal to celebrate. There is a lot to say about delayed gratification sure some of the best accomplishment in our lives we sacrificed and held out for the big enchilada. Allowing yourself to enjoy life during your process keeps you enthused and rejuvenated to maintain your excitement around your goals.

8: START A JOURNAL!

Start a journal. Write down your feelings on paper. Journaling gives you an opportunity to be more expressive and free flowing with what you are feeling at the time. It is different than scheduling your goals in a planner. A journal gives you the opportunity to think through while writing your goals on paper. It becomes a paper trail of our actions and progress. It has an added benefit of meditation. Journaling has a built in accountability factor as well. Journals can be our private joy factor because most journals are private we are more transparent and open and expressive about our goals and dreams.

9: READ A BOOK, LISTEN TO AUDIO OR ATTEND A CONFERENCE!

There are many great books and audio to keep your daily motivation going. Look online for well-known motivational speakers who specialize in motivating and encouraging people to live out their dreams. The more knowledge you get on the subject and reading the inspirational stories you will develop an understanding that you are not alone. This gives you a framework to build up your own motivation. Register for a conference in your area or travel out of town to attend a conference. There is a unique dynamic that goes with attending events a long side of thousands of other people who share the same goals and aspire to be successful as you do. Plug into that synergy.

Conventions and events are designed to keep your motivation and enthusiasm in full swing. However, it is not just enough to get hooked & addicted on the enthusiasm and motivation of a conference you still must learn how to make all the information you learned applicable to your life once you get back to your daily routines.

Attend at least 2 conferences a year and make it a habit of reading a new book every month.

10: DECIDE TO COMMIT!

Have you ever seen someone struggling to make a decision? You will hear them say: "Decisions, Decisions, Decisions!" This catch phrase becomes problematic to the untrained mind. People confuse trying to decide what to do with options on what to do. A decision is a finite resolve to the many options you may have but a decision means to cut off all other paths of your Yes, No or Maybe routes. Rule of thumb, always keep your options open and close your decisions. Funny thing happens when we decide to do something. Guess what? We are more likely to actually do it! Ok don't throw the book away now after this life hack spoiler alert.

Keep reading!

We may not follow through on everything we decide to do but how on earth can we be real about hitting our goals if we have not even decided to do anything?

Make the decision to commit to
bring your motivation into focus. Its
ok we are going to fall off of the
wagon and get off track sometimes.
Life is the up and downs so don't be
so hard on yourself, always find your
strength to dust yourself off and
continue along your path.

Dopamine better known as our "Feel Good Genie in the Bottle" or our pleasure seeking zone. I spoke about a hypothetical pill for motivation well, dopamine would be that pill. Dopamine affects our emotions, our feelings of happy, sad, excited, depressed, enthusiastic, energized and motivated. It is worthy to note our brain processes and stores all pleasure signals whether the source stems from an addictive self-destructive habit or an immensely good satisfying habit such as love in the same suitcase (it packs it all in). Dopamine has even been linked to social media use. You ask how? Studies show many people become depressed after spending too much time on social media. Also there are studies that indicate a dopamine rush with people who tend to excessively post to social media for instant gratification. So be sure to balance your dopamine levels and not spend too much time participating in nonproductive pseudo dopamine rush activities.

Make sure you increase your dopamine levels in a way that supports your healthiest lifestyle.

Motivated people perfect the art of keeping their dopamine levels very high via constructive productive methods. It metaphorically speaking is the drug of life.

Dopamine as stated previously is our body's pleasure hormone found in our brains.

It is our brains neurotransmitter and the key factor to our productivity and motivation.

If you find yourself constantly depressed and unmotivated in life there is a big chance your body's dopamine's levels are low. Look for ways to naturally increase your dopamine levels.

Symptoms of Dopamine Deficiency

Depression

Chronic Boredom

Chronic Fatigue

Lack of Energy

Below are 10 natural creative ways to increase your dopamine levels:

1: Avoid Sugars

2: Exercise

3: Pray ~ Meditate

4: Sleep

5: Massage Therapy

6: Cold Shower

7: Coffee

8: Dance

9: Get some Sun

10: Watch Cartoons

| EAT YOUR MOTIVATION |

When your Motivation is literally
starving to death…..

Your blood sugar levels can easily
impact your mood and energy which
in turn impacts our abilities to make
decisions. If you are not eating
properly you will not feel much like
applying yourself effectively in
reaching your goals. The foods we
eat are very important to our bodies
in particular our brain. The brain is
not the mind. The brain is the
physical part of our body that
houses all of our thoughts, emotions
and mental faculties. The mind is
the most powerful tool we have in
our entire life.

Our cognitive abilities to perceive, imagine, think, reason and our willpower all resides in our mind. We feed our mind via our thoughts and meditation. Many people think the brain is their mind.

Our brain is physical in matter it is the computer that houses the intricate software of the mind.

The brain is very important any imbalance in the brain can severely impact our entire body from our mind to every square inch of our body. The brain requires quality foods, sleep and water. So you want to make sure you are feeding your brain super powerful foods that keep the brain and mind healthy and working in tip-top optimal shape.

Below are 20 of the top foods to eat/drink that impact our motivation.

1: Green Leafy Vegetables

2: Glass of Wine

3: Blueberries

4: Walnuts

5: Yerba Mate Tea

6: Beets

7: Peppermint

8: Pumpkin Seeds

9: Salmon

8: Avocados

9: Celery

10: Oatmeal

11: Extra Virgin Olive Oil

12: Bilberry Extract

13: Sage

14: Spinach

15: Green Tea

16: Sardines

17: Coconut

18: Water

19: Apples

20: Rosemary

| MOTIVATING OILS |

Motivation is essential to Life!

Essential oils have an aromatic molecular compound that can penetrate the blood/brain barrier when applied topically or inhaled. Ageless essential oils have been used therapeutically for years to manage depression, lack of energy and mood swings. Essential oils are known as "adaptogens", because of their unique ability to adapt to the needs of the person in need of therapeutic stress relief.

<u>Essential Oils for Motivation</u>

Peppermint Essential Oil

Rosemary Essential Oil

Holy Basil Essential Oil

Eucalyptus Essential Oil

Lemon Grass Essential Oil

Grapefruit Essential Oil

Bergamot Essential Oil

Marjoram Essential Oil

Ginger Essential Oil

Black Spruce Essential Oil

DAY 1

| CHALLENGES |

Challenges are the rocks that strength lies beneath...Pick up your Rock!

If you want strength don't opt for easy!!! Easy will never be a prerequisite to bigger and great things. Easy never builds enough character, skill, courage and endurance needed for real true growth on your health wealth and fitness journey.

DAY 2

| EXCUSES |

Only people interested in loosing play the excuse game

Your excuse zone is where your goals and results go to die. When you stop using excuses you peel your layers back to reveal your true warrior ready to slay your goals on purpose.

DAY 3

| RESULTS |

*Results are based on a results
driven mindset*

Looking for those results that you never worked for again huh? Let's see, if results grew on trees there would still be lazy people who would never pick the high hanging fruit because they don't want to do the work required

Reach higher!

DAY 4

| SORENESS |

Today I will seek purposeful pain

Yes it hurts until it feels so good to be in your greatest health. Are you afraid of the pain of a great workout? Pain means something is happening. It symbolizes growth which yields physical changes in your mind soul and body. Adopt the mantra Soreness is my only reward and the growth I seek.

DAY 5

| GOD'S GRACE |

You already have God's Grace to run your race

Don't beg God to change your body. He has already provided you the essential blueprints to change every area in your life. Your body, your finances, your relationships, your circumstances all of your life journey requirements are already built in. Pray with Faith!

DAY 6

|PAY DAY|

Life pays you according to your mental currency and self-investment.
Be a Lifepreneuer!

Invest in You! Write the check to yourself eat, pray and exercise your way to your Best Life. Make a living earning your worth. Go to work on yourself everyday pay attention to your bottom line! Your bottom line reflects your level of self- investment.

DAY 7

| WEAKNESS |

Make Strength your Weakness

You can only change and improve what you acknowledge! Identify all areas in your life where you are weak. Being weak is only a weakness if you do not practice or implement strategies to address your short comings. It is ok we all are a work in progress.

DAY 8

| RULES |

Break every rule to reveal your
BEST SELF!

There are no rules when it comes to the pursuit of your goals. You don't have to worry about breaking any rules of nature if it aligns with the Law of Self Preservation.
Then the only rule is Do It!!!

DAY 9

| THINK |

DON'T THINK yourself out of it
THINK yourself into it!

What are you telling yourself on a
daily basis? Why would you talk to
yourself in that manner?
Your thoughts reveal your words!
Your words reveal your mindset!
Your actions reveal your beliefs!

DAY 10

| PERFECT |

Perfect is spelled DONE!

Waiting on perfect timing is simply

wasting your time in the Now!

We look for perfect conditions in

our life the perfect mate, body, job,

moment, perfect time to start or stop

You can never go back in time or

predict any future circumstances

you may encounter so

Live in the Now!

DAY 11

| DREAM BODY |

Your dream body is waiting on you to wake up and take action!

Stop Dreaming!

Stop Wishing!

Stop Hoping!

Stop Praying!

Start Doing!

Wake up and take Action!

DAY 12

| TODAY |

I will put one foot in front of the other and make the most of each day

Today is all we have!
Stop believing in yesterday and counting on tomorrow! Yesterday is money spent. Tomorrow is money pending that hasn't hit the bank yet.
Today is Payday!
Hit Pay Dirt Now!

DAY 13

| MENTAL QUICK SAND |

Your thoughts are reaching for
a lifesaver to get you out of
your mental quick sand

Get rid of all your negative thinking!
Negative thinking is the quicksand
that devours your dreams and goals.
Stop the struggle of a negative mind
and immediately focus on your goals
and execute your plan.

DAY 14

| REPETITION |

Think ...Speak... Focus ...
Apply... Repeat...

Habits are the result of repeatedly doing things over and over. When we think positive constructive thoughts, and recite it and speak it over and over you train your mind to get the results you want.

DAY 15

|DAY ONE'S|

The Power of One

Every Start has a Day 1
Every Result started at Day 1
A New Year is a Day 1
Your Day 1 Starts your Journey
1 Day at a time equals Forever

DAY 16

| HALFWAY |

*Halfway there is far better than
all the way No where*

Halfway is the middle ground of progress. The seed(s) that were planted at the start of your journey is what lies beneath growing your hard work and the fruit of your harvest.

DAY 17

| GAME OF LIFE |

Get in the game of Life!
Life is not youth kickball
pick yourself first!

Don't think twice about who never picked you for their team in the past. Its ok they never knew your potential and how great you were. Their loss! Now you are in charge of the selection process, you have full ownership of Team You!

DAY 18

| YOUR VOICE |

*"I AM" living in my
highest thought vibration*

The 1st most powerful tool in your arsenal is "Your Mind" the 2nd most powerful tool is "Your Voice: command, declare and affirm your Best Life! You are reaching your goals and living your highest quality of life through every thought and word uttered.

DAY 19

| COMPLAINERS |

Complainers always "Lose" however, they just don't "Lose Weight"

Don't develop the bad habit of complaining. The only rewards of complaining are recycled bad results. Complaining waters every excuse waiting to sprout as a weed to kill your aspirations and goals.

DAY 20

| IT'S YOU! |

It's not the T-Shirt Or the Sweat pants
Guess who? It's YOU!

The T-shirt sweat pants and sneakers may enhance your motivation but, "You" are your own motivator. Self-Motivation is an important tool on your journey in life and getting things done. Lose all the external trappings and realize your inner fortitude.

DAY 21

|EXCEPTIONAL|

Feel Like Quitting? It's Normal
Don't Be Normal!
Be Exceptional!

Be Exceptional!
Keep your word especially with
yourself. Practice what you Speak!
Create daily habits that break every
excuse that leads to quitting.

DAY 22

| JUST GOD |

God is your biggest cheerleader... Come off the bench of life and hit your free throws

When your road gets rough all you need is to realign with God's Perfect Will over your Life. God gives us Strength, Clarity, Peace and the Will Power to sustain us on every step of our journey.

DAY 23

| MIRROR REFLECTION |

The mirror reflects only what
you choose to see
Look within for real deep
reflection

It's fine not to like everything that reflects back at us in the mirror However, always love your reflection! Life gives us many opportunities for self- improvement and self-love.

DAY 24

| PATIENCE IS A VIRTUE |

Stay out of the emergency room be patient with yourself

An ounce of patience is worth every drip drop of the process. Results are tied to commitment and consistency that leads to permanent changes in our lives. Do not rush away your process with trying to find the shortcuts. You will not arrive earlier than your results. Results equal your estimated time of arrival.

DAY 25

| HABITS |

Become a Habit Junkie!
Habits are the best junk food for
the soul

All life has polarity.
Good habits are hard to make!
Bad habits are hard to break!
Habits will form either way, so
choose your hard or choose your
easy.
The choice is ultimately yours!

DAY 26

| THE COURSE |

Own your process without worrying about your exit

Never abandoned your course! There will be many tempting exits along the way. The finish and done exits may be 25 miles or 500 miles to go. The distance does not matter! Gas up, kick the tires put on your favorite song and enjoy the ride. Just keep going!

DAY 27

Waiting for a perfect time is like waiting in line for the sake of waiting.
You will always end up with nothing!

Don't get stuck in "The Perfect". The Perfect is that sunken place. Get glued to habit forming daily changes. The everyday incremental improvements we make form perfect habits.

DAY 28

Replace negative thoughts with daily positive affirmations. Your Life reflects what you affirm daily

Affirm who you are everyday
starting with the great "I AM"
"I Am" Enlighted
"I Am" Determined
"I Am" Powerful
"I Am" Successful
"I Am" made in his Image!

DAY 29

|PAY ATTENTION|

Your attention will either EARN you the lifestyle you DESIRE or COST you the lifestyle you WANT

Pay attention to what you are thinking! Where your attention goes, your energy flows so focus your time, attention and energy only on goal oriented thoughts that visually and physically move you closer to your goals.

DAY 30

| HARD WORK |

Desire starts the fire...
Motivation fans the flame...
Heat comes from hard work...

Nobody likes hard work! We all would love for life to get easier. The thing is easy never precedes real work. If the work is easy there is no room for challenges to grow, stretch and pull us into our greatest potential.
Our challenges become our testimony.

DAY 31

| MASTER KEY |

If you ask "Can I do it?" You
have lost before you started
If you command "I can do it"
You unlock your door

If it has been done, you can do it!
If it has never been done you can do
that too! We wait a lifetime for
doors to magically open without a
slightest twist of the door knob. The
real truth, some doors are just not
our door to open. We all hold the
master key.

DAY 32

| WISHING ON A STAR |

Transform your wishing into working
Don't have a wishful thinking Blueprint

Wishful thinking is only good in fairy tales and blowing out candles on a birthday cake. Wishing on a star to change your daily habits will never change your lifestyle. The universe only brings forth deliberate intentions.

DAY 33

| FEAR |

Most fears are a result of the unknown. There are two roads on your journey of Life Faith .vs. Fear.

If you looked up the word Fear, most people's picture would be displayed. Take your picture out of the lineup. Make sure your picture is under the "Got it done!" folder! Don't allow fear to block your blessings!

DAY 34

|SAY IT! DO IT!|

You can only measure what you completed!

Don't say what didn't work!
Identify what you did or did not do
and make a plan, outline strategies,
prioritize and stay focused.
Saying something does not work,
will never replace doing what it takes
to get the job done!

DAY 35

| CONSISTENT |

Consistency is the flower that grows in the dark patiently waiting to be revealed

Each day gifts us with built in consistency. It's God's way of saying "Ok time to do it again!" The challenge is our ability to master our daily thoughts over and over to bring about change.

DAY 36

| ENOUGH |

The POWER lies within
You are more than ENOUGH!

You are enough you don't need a
step counter
You don't need a gadget!
You don't need the latest app!
You don't need technology!
Your mind is God's greatest
invention!

DAY 37

| PASSION |

Good Health is the Passion and Art of Living well

Make health your number one passion and priority. Become mentally, emotionally and physically determined to live the healthiest Life ever! Connect to your inner passions! Brighten and excite this world with your True Authenticity!

DAY 38

| HOPE |

Hoping is a one way ticket to a
Shipwrecked Island
Doing is a seat in first class to
Paradise Island

Reaching your health and fitness goals will require more than the notion of hope. It will require fueling your hope with action(s) getting in the trenches, knocking down procrastination, ditching the excuses and bad habits.

DAY 39

| TOUGH |

Mental toughness is the training ground for every fight in life!
Get in the trenches fight the right battle

Your physical body will never be stronger than your mental toughness.

That last rep was not because your body is stronger than your mind, It is because your mind said you can do it!, and you did it!

DAY 40

| FALL DOWN |

Fall down 100 times
Get back up 100,000 times
Never be afraid to fall
be afraid of staying down

Falling down is a part of the process. Falling may hurt you may require a band aid or even stitches. The bruise or cut will take time to heal. Bruises fade and the scar leaves you with a reminder that your fall did not stop you from getting back up one more time.

DAY 41

| TIME |

Time is never up on a changed MIND!

It's time for you to make a decision that will transform your life forever. Decide to be healthy a clock can never reflect a moment in time. Your power to make a decision in a split second beats the ticks and tocks of a clock. Your mind is a clock that is always set to "Now"!

DAY 42

| WORRY |

Never worry if you will reach a goal(s)…Worry if you never set any goals in Life

There is absolutely nothing to worry about when you decide to make positive changes in your life. Boldly declare your goals, write them down, plain and execute them daily. Modify where and when necessary. No time for worrying. It is done!

DAY 43

| THOUGHT |

Don't put more thought into what you will EAT Over what you feed your MIND! Thought is the starving appetite that gets fed first

Your every thought is directly related to an outer manifestation in your life.

Thoughts rule the universe!

Feed your mind before feeding your body and grow and prosper in the right areas of your life!

DAY 44

| GIFT |

Exercise all of your gifts Faith, Mind and Purpose

Don't give yourself a choice to
exercise!
Give yourself the gift of exercise!
There is a difference!
Exercise is the gift with the prettiest
red bow under the tree
Unwrap your gift of exercise daily!

DAY 45

| SHAPE |

*A STRONG BODY will keep you
in great Shape
A STRONG MIND will shape
your WORLD!*

Shaping the body is the easy part.
Reshaping your thought pattern is
the most challenging part.
A strong mind is the muscle that
nobody ever sees that forms and
shapes our world.

DAY 46

| INVEST |

Investing in self are your personal reward credits to a free and ABUNDANT LIFE!

Take the wonder out of how can I do this? Invest in accomplishing what needs to be done!
Investing in self yields the highest Return on Investment in life!

DAY 47

There is no light at the end of the tunnel. The only light that exist is deep inside you is 'Your Why"

Why have you decided to change your life? Keep your why front and center it will light your path when your journey gets dim and sometimes dark. When the lights go out, when people leave and when you're all alone in your solitude,
God knows your "Why".

DAY 48

| EXPENSE |

Dreams are costly!
Thoughts are the currency that
purchases dreams, goals and the
lifestyle you desire

A thought is your cheapest
overhead expense to attract
prosperity and good will and yields a
life well lived. It pays more dividends
than a dreamed lottery win!

DAY 49

| SCORE |

Don't play the sidelines
Don't be a spectator in your
own life, run up the score don't
let life win

Set a goal drop kick the ball over
the goal line and score in life.
Realize you are the franchise player.
The game needs you!

DAY 50

| OPPORTUNITY |

Every day is an opportunity waiting to connect you with your higher purpose

Every day is the most missed opportunity to pursue your dreams with purpose. Each day gets overlooked, misused, wasted and taken for granted. Opportunity does not always knock it appears every day at sunrise.

DAY 51

| UNSTOPPABLE |

Your Mind makes you
UNSTOPPABLE
Your Mind can also STOP YOU!

The only thing that can stop you is
death. Since you are reading this
you are still unstoppable!
There is still enough time on the
clock.
Go get it!

DAY 52

| TRANSFORM |

Thoughts transform expectation and beliefs into tangible things

Real transformation is not visible via eyesight alone. Mindset changes equals physical & lifestyle changes! People will only see the canvas of your life but never see the paint brush that exist in your mind's eye.

DAY 53

Keep running...Keep working...Keep doing...Keep believing....Keep going!

Starting and finishing has nothing to do with the race of Life. Don't rush your life away. There is no finish line that exist in life! There is only "The Dash" between our born date and the date of death. Train for your dash, not a finish line.

DAY 54

| PROUD |

*Celebrate your small victories
each day*

Be proud of where you are today!
No matter if it's your Day 1
Nobody ever starts at Day 100!
Nobody finishes before they start!
"It just happened overnight!!" said
nobody who has worked for their
success in life.

DAY 55

| TRY |

Trying is failure's kryptonite

Trying is preceded by a decision!
Tying is aligning with the master
thought you hold in your mind.
A decision precedes all success!
Decide then Do It!

DAY 56

| GREATNESS |

Greatness is nothing more than baby steps to a choreographed dance

Greatness is embedded in all of our DNA! Unlocking your greatness is established in creating consistent daily good habits.

DAY 57

|CONTROL|

You are the remote that changes the channel in your Life

Taking full control of your life requires controlling what you:

Think!

Speak!

Do!

DAY 58

| DISCIPLINE |

*Your decision to commit is
what feeds and nourishes the
starvation of your goals*

Discipline happens in 3 words:
Decide To Commit!
Discipline is the strong talk & tough
love we display in our actions when
our minds try to wimp out of doing
what we said we would do.

DAY 59

| BREAKTHROUGH |

Your breakthrough is looking for you, and is necessary to shift your entire perspective of life.

Your breakthroughs happen at your breaking point! Either you will rise to the occasion or, you will take a seat in the backrow and the understudy gets the leading role.

DAY 60

| RELATIVELY FIT |

Put Fit into its proper
perspective

Fit is not only about fitting those
favorite size 8 jeans
That looked so nice on your frame
at 20 years old,
Life is about being Holistically
Healthy and Fit on
all levels and in every area of your
life.

DAY 61

| FEAR |

Take the fear out of not knowing and know what it feels like to   Win Big in Life!

Fear is the number one killer!
Fear kills dreams, fear kills goals,
fear kills belief, fear kills progress,
fear kills change, fear kills
transformation.
Ultimately, fear kills living
abundantly.

DAY 62

| CIRCUMSTANCES |

Conquer your Circumstances with Commitment Consistency Control and Change

Your current circumstances don't equal your end result!
Your end results are a culmination of your mindset, commitment, habits, self- control & consistency that leads to effective and permanent change.

DAY 63

| HURT |

The regret of a No Pain Lifestyle

The pain associated with the regret of not moving past your fears hurts more than the hardest workout. Achieving the things you set out to do is the painkiller for life's regrets. Do not live in the shadow of regrets and I should've could've done that if I tried.

DAY 64

| GUILTY |

What you think in private is on public display

Release your private thoughts of the guilt and shame for not achieving all you set out to do.
Yesterday will never come around again and today is all you need for a fresh New Start!

DAY 65

| CHANGE |

A moment of instant change can surpass years of meticulous planning

Don't spend all your waking hours talking, planning and setting goals to change your life. Change happens at the speed of thought which travels faster than the speed of light! A decision to change is fastest way to change your life.

DAY 66

| TRUE INSPIRATION |

Close your eyes
stop looking outside of yourself
it is called "Inspiration"

Inspiration can come from many places. The best inspiration resides inside all of us. True Inspiration is when we are able to be vulnerable with our most authentic self to serve our highest purpose for those who are need of inspiration.

DAY 67

|EXCUSES|

There is no currency in the universe for excuses the quicker you lose all your excuses the wealthier you become

Take every excuse to the bank how much does it pay? Zero!
99.9 percent of failure comes from excuse making mentality.
Hard work pays residuals in every area of your life.

DAY 68

| FORTUNE |

Living an inspired life is PAID IN FULL

You hit the lottery every day you wake up! Now go spend your massive fortune on the things money can't buy. Life provides us real wealth in health, love, inspiration, laugher, kindness, compassion and forgiveness.

DAY 69

| HIT HARD |

*Life is a hard hitter, make
every punch count towards
living your best life*

Life hits harder than any workout so
train harder to absorb the blows.
You will not win every fight in your
lifetime, nobody is immune to the
life's ups and downs.
Resolve to fight! Stay in the battle!

DAY 70

|DETERMINATION|

Reap the rewards of results
from the seed of determination

You can't say you want it but
unwilling to do what it takes
Stick with the program stay with the
process. Results and determination
go hand in hand!

DAY 71

| THE HERO INSIDE |

You are the hero you seek waiting for the signal to come to your own rescue!

Heroes don't fly out of the clear blue sky or run into a phone booth to save you when we are in dire straits. Sorry to spoil the plot. Our ultimate responsibility is to save ourselves!

DAY 72

| DESTINY |

You are destined to do whatever it is you set your mind to do!

God's gives us free will. Your destiny is who you decide to be! Not what you decide to do! The person you decide to be has the God given right to follow any dream & reach any goal in life irrespective to others opinions and judgements.

DAY 73

| REAFFIRM |

*Repeat your dreams and goals
like you recited your ABCs*

Reaffirm your dreams daily!
Repetitive thoughts and words are
the magic source that aligns us with
the vast abundance of this universe.
Speak your dreams and goals out
loud, write them down, hold the vision
clear, meditate, bless them up and do
the work!

DAY 74

| STRUGGLE |

What you think consistently and dwell on shows up in two different ways Struggles .vs. Success

The struggle is all in your mind command your thoughts! A conscious thought pattern aligns you with your vision daily. It is your mental compass to guide you in the right direction towards your goals. Allow your vision the insight of positive thinking.

DAY 75

| WISHES |

Wishes are our goals and dreams waiting for a ride to manifest in real life. The vehicle is work!

Replace wishful thinking with an impeccable work ethic. Work is the bridge that connects wishing & fruition. Cross the bridge in your mind before you physically get there. Never be afraid of bridges that bring you out of your comfort zone.

DAY 76

| OBSTACLES |

*The biggest obstacles in life are
those roadblocks, speed bumps,
detours & stop signs that are
continuously in your mind*

There will always be obstacles in life
on your path and journey.
Just make sure you are not the
obstacle blocking your own dreams.
Simply get up out your own way!

DAY 77

| ACHIEVING |

The mind has to conceive &
believe in order to achieve it.
The mind is your real life vision
board

You will achieve all that you believe.
You must hold the daily conscious
thought of your goals
You must visualize!
You must meditate! You must first
see it in your mind's eye

DAY 78

| SURRENDER |

The art of surrendering is a
powerful force of healing

Surrendering is a strength that
never gets the credit it deserves.
Surrendering takes courage and
faith in knowing that what we can't
do in this physical world. God is so
able in the spiritual realm for our
super natural healing and
breakthrough.

DAY 79

| WILL YOU? |

You have ultimate control the moment you give up your control your willpower depletes

Will you do it?
Will you let another goal slide?
Will you let another year pass?
Will you continue with all your excuses? Only you can answer that question! Can you do it? Yes you can!
Now what are you going to do?
You are in control of your will power!

DAY 80

|GOALS|

*Reaching our goals shows us
our abilities to tap into our
power deep within*

Goals allow us to practice the art of
self-improvement and personal
development & growth to prevent
ourselves from becoming complacent
and comfortable with living a regular
existence in life.
Goals give our lives greater
purpose.

DAY 81

| HATE |

There is no room for hate when you extend yourself self-love

Never hate anything about yourself. Hate makes us bitter and unreceptive to appreciating what God has allowed us to be in this world.
Change the things you wish to improve about yourself. Do not hate yourself! Hating leaves no room for your best self!

DAY 82

| CELEBRATE |

*Celebrate often and reward
yourself with setting new goals*

Get used to hearing You Did It!!!
Over and Over and Over and
Over again.
Never miss a chance to celebrate
your accomplishments you deserve it
for a job well done! Congratulations
in advance to all of your many
accomplishments!

DAY 83

| REPETITION |

Repeating thoughts, words and actions create change

If necessity is the mother of invention then surely repetition is the mother of all learning. We have created deep set paradigms in our lives. Repetition makes the mind pay attention to what we want our brains to remember. If you want to change your life intentionally say, do and behave in a perpetual state of constant repetition.

DAY 84

| SUCCESS |

Success in 3 words:
Practice being Great!

Success is nothing more than never missing opportunities to practice the art of mastering ordinary task. Practice is as close to perfect as we get. Great people are not born they practice their craft and master their thought process.

DAY 85

| DESIRE |

Transform your wishful desire
into fueled passion with
premium grade work

Desire is nothing more than an unfueled dream. What happens when your car runs low on fuel? You go pump more fuel to keep your vehicle going. Our dreams are fueled with passion and work or all we have are broken down dreams on the road of life.

DAY 86

| WIN |

Winning is not everything says the person who lost weight

Sometimes losing is more beneficial than winning. Weight loss of course is one of those times. This is when being a loser is 1st place. You can stand to lose a few other than weight. Lose those bad daily habits, poor mental conditioning and self-doubting.

DAY 87

| COUNT |

Don't count your steps
make every step on your
journey count!

Stop counting your steps!
Stop counting calories!
Stop counting pounds on the scale!
Stop counting the minutes on the
treadmill!
Start counting on Yourself!

DAY 88

| BELIEVE |

Learn to affirm!
Affirmations align us with
thoughts that grow into our
core values and beliefs that
become our foundation of life!

Stop believing in the person you
think you are not!
Start believing in the person you
Affirm Daily!

DAY 89

| WARNING! |

WARNING!! You are becoming a better you

Believe in yourself!
Invest in yourself!
Work on your goals daily!
Be Consistent!
Be Intentional!
Be Deliberate!
Be Better!

DAY 90

| REGRETS |

Regrets typically are not found reaching new heights. Regrets are found looking up at missed opportunities to go higher

You will never find regrets in reaching your goals. The biggest regrets in life are the goals left alone in the dark, the goals you eloquently reasoned yourself from pursuing because you were too busy or too afraid of your own success.

DAY 91 *BONUS

| REAL WORTH |

You are worth all your time and effort you invest in your personal development

Stop what you are doing and repeat out loud

"I Am Worth It"

While smiling and envisioning yourself reaching all your goals and how it feels to be a winner in life

Repeat 10 Times!!!

DAY 92 *BONUS

| LIME TO A LEMON |

Use your disappointments as opportunities to CLEANSE your life

When life throws you lemons
Make it a cleanse day!

DAY 93 *BONUS

| DISTRACTIONS |

Become laser focused on your goals distractions are outside of the realm of the needle's eye

Get crystal clear on your goals
Develop a plan of action
Adjust your goal(s) lens daily.

DAY 94 *BONUS

|SACRED RITUALS|

Greet each day with a Good morning prayer before your feet hit the ground.

Practice the art of perfecting rituals that sustain your daily habits. Cultivate and nourish everyday thoughts and actions in order to achieve the lifestyle you dreamed.

DAY 95 *BONUS

|HOLISTIC|

Integrative health happens in 3 words "Mind Body Soul"

You will not reach any level of

success without incorporating

"Mind Body and Soul Wellness"

Do not focus on one without

incorporating the others.

DAY 96 *BONUS

| SPEAK LOUD |

SPEAK ABUNDANT LIFE!!!

Words unspoken are goals and
dreams deferred
Give the universe explicit directions!

DAY 97 *BONUS

| MENTAL CARDIO |

Brain Train
Physical endurance is your
mind on a treadmill

Your mind has to be at the finish line way before your body starts the race. The body gets tired when the mind is exhausted make sure you are doing those sets and reps keep the mind strong ready for the marathon of life.

DAY 98 *BONUS

| GOAL HORTICULTURE |

Water brings good seeds to life.
Plant your seeds and give them
water, food, good attention and
respect the growth cycle

Your follow through waters the
seeds of: Get it Done! & Finished!
Everything in life has a process of
growth. All forms of life have their
respective gestation period.
Sow and Grow!

DAY 99 *BONUS

| FAILURE |

Don't be the "I" in Failure

Do not believe you are protecting yourself from failure by not going for it & giving it your all. Low expectation of self never leads to God's master plan for your life. There is no failure in setting goals, working on your goals and believing in yourself.

DAY 100 *BONUS

| COMMIT |

Commit to Life!

If You Can Commit To
100 Days
You Can Commit To
365 Days
If you Can Commit To
365 Days
You Can Commit To
An Ultimate Health and Wellness
Lifestyle Forever!

|CERTIFICATE OF COMPLETION|

*****CONGRATULATIONS!*****

____

SIGN YOUR NAME HERE

HAS SUCCESSFULLY COMPLETED
THE 90-DAY INNER MOTIVATION
FIERCE FACTOR CHALLANGE